TABLE OF CONTENTS

Introduction

Ever heard of essential oils and aromatherapy? Wondering what they are? Well, essential oils are natural, pure and healthy oils that are extracted from the naturally growing herbs and plants in the forest, garden or as shrubs. It is important to note that these plants and herbs possess medicinal properties that stimulates and boosts the natural healing ability of the body. These oils come in their concentrated form thus requiring to be added into a career oil such as olive oil and almond oil while diluted in the right proportions if to be used by children. Essential oils are ideal for aromatherapy, which is a natural process that ensures health and wellness by the use of the oils.

In this site, we have provided enough information about the essential oils, their different types, how to use them, how to make them, the ailments and situations in which they should be used. The oils are safe for human use as well as with pets and around the home for different tasks. Browse through to find adequate and helpful information about essential oils and their benefits to your body. In a hurry and you want to scan through? Access the FAQ section for specific brief and simplified information in the form of questions and answers.

Benefits of Essential Oils regarding anti-aging and Beauty

Essential oils have anti-aging and beauty properties that make them varied for use by people across the gender and age brackets. As much as everyone wishes to remain beautiful, no one likes the appearance that comes with the advanced age. This is because the face is the first part of the body that meets other people's eyes; thus when invaded by wrinkles, pimples and spots it is not attractive. Essential oils act on the skin enhancing the natural beauty in an individual and slowing down the aging process. Unlike other beauty and anti-aging products, these oils are derived from plants and processed without adding any chemicals that can harm the skin or the body. Therefore, the oils do not cause a bleaching effect, and they enhance health and wellness in the individual.

However, it should be noted that these oils are extracted from plants through a distillation process. This makes them pure and highly concentrated. It is therefore advisable to consider diluting them with other pure oils such as olive, castor or almond oil instead of using them directly on the skin. This helps in providing the best results, making the skin smooth, soft, young and beautiful.

Skin type that requires use of essential oils

Dry skin

Disturbed by a dry skin? Well, essential oils are a viable solution required to make the skin smooth and soft. Dry skin is caused by inadequate oil or moisture necessary to lubricate the skin. Though this can depend on the type of body lotion one uses, there are some skin types that become dry a few hours after the lotion is applied. However, the oils act on the skin, soothing and keeping it relaxed while moisturizing it all the day. These oils do not make the skin appear oily or excessively shinny, but soft even in harsh weather.

Cracking skin

The essential oils have a long history of healing the cracking skin. Apart from preventing formation of more cracks on the facial skin, the oils have antiseptic characteristics that protect the body from infections through the present cracks. After a period of using these natural oils, the skin becomes smooth, soft and without marks on the areas previously cracked.

Acne affected skin

The presence of acne on the facial skin makes one uncomfortable due to the trail of spots they leave on the skin. In addition, they make the skin very sensitive, sometimes becoming itchy and oily. Cystic acne is normally caused by bacterial infection on the skin leading to eruption of pimples on the face. The essential oils are effective in treatment of acne as they eliminate the bacteria present bringing about healing. Also, the oils soothe the affected areas of the skin hence preventing itchiness that may lead to openings for more infections. Once the acne is cleared, the oils leave the skin smooth without a trace of spots through their cleansing properties.

Oily skin

When the skin secretes excessive oil, the skin of the face becomes very oily. Due to a busy schedule one may not have enough time to wash the face during the day. The oily skin becomes a favorable home for pathogens that cause skin diseases. Use of essential oils is ideal for oily skin as they help in getting rid of the excessive oil secreted from the skin.

Top essential oils for aging skin and beauty

Clary sage essential oil

The Clary serge oil is known for its multiple uses in the skincare process. The oil delays the aging process on the skin by making fine lines and wrinkles present on the facial skin smooth. It provides amazing results when used with skin moisturizers that make the skin fresh, soft and healthy. This natural oil also helps in making the pores of the skin tight. The Clary sage essential oil is also best for dry skin.

Grapefruit essential oil

This essential oil is derived from the seeds of the grapes that have antioxidant properties and are full of vitamin E. The oil provides the best results in healing of skin that has been damaged. Thus, it can be used on cracking skin or one effected by acne. In addition, the vitamin E present keeps the skin young and beautiful as it slows down the aging process hence preventing formation of lines and wrinkles associated with old age.

Lemon essential oils

The natural oils derived from the lemon plant are best for oily skins and those affected by acne. The oil has the antiseptic properties that heals and protects the skin from infections. It can be used along other essential oils.

Myrrah natural oil

This essential oil is known for its antioxidant characteristics that help in restoring the damaged skin. The oil keeps the facial skin moisturized while smoothening out the wrinkles. This brings out a smooth, soft and young healthy skin.

Jasmine essential oil

The jasmine oil is ideal for dry and cracking skin. This is because it soothes, moisturizes and relaxes the skin. It provides great results when mixed with other oils such as the olive oil. It can also be used together with facial lotions that are not mixed with chemicals that bleach the skin.

Geranium essential oil

This natural oil is ideal for all type of facial skin. The geranium oil helps in enhancing blood circulation within the skin as an organ hence ensuring adequate moisture. This makes the oil best for dry and cracking skin as well as the oily skin. When used along other skin moisturizers, the oil provides the best results.

Orange essential oil

The orange natural oil has both antiseptic and moistening effects on the skin. This makes it the best solution for a dry skin as well as an aging one. In this case, the oil makes the skin smooth by getting rid of the wrinkles present on the skin hence making one young and beautiful.

Conclusion

The essential oils provide the desired results when used on the skin going through the aging process and the one suffering from different attacks. The oils act on the dry, oily, acne affected and wrinkled skin that takes the beauty away from an individual. The essential oils keep the skin moisturized, smooth and soft thus young, beautiful and healthy.

DIY AROMATHERAPY AND ESSENTIAL OILS

DIY aromatherapy and essential oils is a topic that is important as it addresses important issues about the health of the entire family. The essential oils are tapped from the different plants and used while pure and natural. Depending on the type of the plant the oil can be extracted from the stem, leaves, fruits or roots. These oils are part of aromatherapy recipe that is successfully done by use of the natural flavor, scent and properties in the oils to provide the desired effects. They are the best substitutes for over the counter medication as they work towards boosting the natural healing process of the body. They are also best used as beauty products and anti-aging agents that keep the skin smooth, moisturized and soft while delaying the aging process that has a great impact on the skin. Essential oils have proven to be good agents for home cleaning and freshness in the house as well. In addition, the oils are great in protecting and healing pets from related diseases.

Must have essential oils for DIY aromatherapy

When purchasing the essential oils, a budget should be made carefully. This entails identifying the purpose of the oils and which types are ideal. Here are some of the oils that must be in the list for the DIY aromatherapy.

Lavender essential oil

The lavender natural oil is one of the must have essential oils. The oil is known for its soothing effect on the body. It acts on the nerve and brain cells as well as the skin leading to relaxation and calmness. It also induces sleep when taken slightly before bedtime hence ensuring a deep sleep. These properties make the oil ideal for stress and depression related issues.

In addition, this oil is effective as a beauty product. When applied on the skin, it enhances natural beauty, it smoothens out the wrinkles, fine lines, spots and scars present on the skin. It is also a great lip balm that protects the lips from cracking while facilitating healing of the same. The unique aspect of this oil is that it is safe for use on children especially for diaper rash.

Lemon essential oil

Lemon natural oil is used in a wide range of needs. It can be taken orally, inhaled or applied on the skin to provide the desired results. Lemon oil facilitates digestion for people who are prone to constipation and other digestive related issues. This oil acts on the skin protecting it from infections and hastening the natural healing process. When inhaled, the lemon oil clears the sinuses, throat and chest in case of a flu and common cold. In case of depression, anxiety and stress, the lemon oil should be used for bathing, along with in tea or water and as spray in the room at night to bring about deep relaxation to the muscles, brain and nerves.

In addition, lemon essential oil is used as a cleaning agent in the house. It helps in washing of dishes full of grease while providing a shinny deep cleansing to the utensils. It is also ideal for floor and bench cleaning especially in the kitchen and play room for the kids. A special aspect of this oil is that it helps in keeping the flies and other insects out of the house.

Tea Tree essential oil

Tea tree essential oil is an effective antimicrobial agent. It is ideal for aromatherapy as well as for other cleaning tasks around the house. This oil is among the top beauty enhancing natural products that clears marks from the skin without causing any bleaching effect. When used in aromatherapy, the oil protects the skin from infections as it possesses antimicrobial properties. One can also add a few drops into the bathtub for a good soak for a more relaxed body.

Apart from being effective on the body, this essential oil can be sprayed on the benches and floor especially in the kitchen as a disinfectant. This is because it kills many strains of germs.

Peppermint essential oil

Peppermint oil is popular for its ability to soothe away pain and kill disease causing bacteria. These properties make it ideal for aromatherapy. It is a good replacement for pain killers prescribed over the counter as it numbs the pain. For those suffering from diseases resulting from inflammation such as arthritis, this oil is a must have all the time as it acts as an anti-inflammatory agent. For those affected by extreme weather during summer, a massage with peppermint oil provides the most refreshing cooling effect in the body.

Peppermint essential oil can be mixed with carrier oil such as coconut oil and then used to massage or rub the body muscles hence eliminating pain and soothing the body. However, the eyes and other mucus membranes should be protected from direct contact with peppermint as it can cause irritation.

Eucalyptus essential oil

The power of natural eucalyptus oil is based on its scent and antimicrobial properties. This makes it ideal for help with respiratory system issues such as the common cold and flu that causes nasal and chest congestion. This oil is used in aromatherapy in different ways. For example the oil is inhaled to help in clearing the blocked chest and respiratory tract. In addition, the oil is sprayed into the room in which the person suffering from flu is living especially at night to facilitate easy breathing. It is also rubbed on the chest to ease congestion.

Due to its ability to kill germs, the eucalyptus natural oil is used as a cleaning agent for utensils, the floor and bed linen. This helps in ensuring good health for everyone in the household.

Conclusion

DIY aromatherapy becomes effective when done using the essential oils that are natural, pure and potent. The oils can be used during a bath by adding them in the shower shampoo, inhaled, taken with water or tea, as disinfectant through spraying and as beauty product. The essential oils always provide the desired results in every session of aromatherapy.

Essential Oils and Weight Loss

Essential oils are part of the weight loss plan as they provide excellent results. The oils offers a natural remedy to lose weight instead of using chemical pills that leads to weight loss while causing undesirable effects in the body. However, it is advisable to combine the use of the oils with healthy diet and exercises for best results. The role of the essential oils in the weight loss process is to boost the energy, mood and action of the diet and exercises towards losing the desired amount of weight within the desired period of time. This is because the essential oils can be taken with the major meals and used for toning the body after sweaty exercises. However, the essential oils are ideal in controlling the appetite through their fragrance hence enhancing the ability to adhere to the diet plan that leads to significant weight loss.

Factors to consider when using essential oils for weight loss

The following factors should be considered for a successful use of essential oils for weight loss purposes.

Availability of variety of essential oils

It is advisable to check on the availability of a wide variety of essential oils to use for weight loss purposes. In this case, you can identify about three to five different types of the essential oils to be used during the day. This is because the body can adapt to the smell of a certain essential oil if it is used alone for several days consistently. Remember that smelling the fragrance in the essential oils controls the appetite hence slowing down the desire to indulge in eating at the time outside the planned feeding schedule. Therefore, having a variety of the essential oils in the car, house and place of work boosts adherence to meal time plans as they help in avoiding the temptation of eating.

Effectiveness of the oils

The reaction of the body towards the smell of each of the essential oils varies from one person to the other. Thus, it is important to identify the set of oils that works best for you in terms of delaying gratification for feeding. It is advisable to have a test phase in which you experiment on different types of the oils hence coming up with a set of about five that are effective.

Compatibility

Essential oils are natural and pure extracts from the plants. However, they are highly concentrated with a strong scent. When using the oils for weight loss purposes, you will be required to smell directly through the nose. Some of these oils have been found to cause some burning sensations in the nostrils for some people when smelt directly. Therefore, it is important to try out the available essential oils in order to find out if they are compatible with your body.

Mode of using them

It is advisable to determine the mode of using the essential oil for the purposes of weight loss. It should be noted that though the primary mode of using the oils for weight loss is through the smell, others can be taken with the meals in a healthy diet to boost immunity in the body for better adjustment to weight loss. In addition, other oils can be used for bathing after workout sessions in the gym with the aim of relaxing the tensed muscles bringing about wellness. Thus, once the mode is identified, it is possible to choose the ideal essential oils for use.

Top essential oils to be used for weight loss purposes

Bergamot essential oils

Bergamot is among the most effective essential oils for weight loss. Its action is based on its ability to eliminate emotional stress that accounts for the highest percentage of overeating leading to massive weight gain. This natural oil works on the endocrine system bringing about calmness and well being that replaces the stress present. This oil delivers the best results if used together with lavender oil that boosts its action. To use this oil, you need to have a handkerchief and pour on it about two to three drops of the bergamot oil and inhale deeply. The inhaled fragrance works in the body system bringing about relaxation.

Sandalwood essential oil

The essential oil derived from the sandalwood works on the body system bringing about a sense of wellness and relaxation. This essential oil is known for its action on the brain cell that boosts its ability to resist desire to feed in excess. This allows one to adhere to the weight loss diet program while ensuring a feeling of serenity in an individual. This gives way to weight loss when combined with a healthy diet and exercise. The route of administration is through inhalation.

Peppermint essential oil

Peppermint is another potent essential oil that is taken orally while mixed with water or tea which should be taken slightly before meals. In addition, it should be taken through inhalation of some drops poured out on a handkerchief. This natural oil acts on both the brain cells and the stomach hence being ideal to be used in a weight loss process. In this case, the peppermint oil brings about a feeling of having a full stomach hence no need to feed in excess. Also, it stimulates the cells of the brain hence sending messages of calmness that eliminates emotional stress. The oil is ideal for effective digestion, preventing stomach issues hence facilitating adequate absorption of the healthy diet. All these aspects enhance weight loss as desired.

Grapefruit essential oil

When the fatty acids in the body are released into the blood stream, they are broken down into energy hence preventing accumulation of fats that leads to weight gain. Taking the grapefruit essential oil aids in an increase in dissolving of the fatty acids into the blood stream where they are changed into energy. This action is facilitated by the presence of limonene in the grapefruit oil. The oil is taken through inhalation or orally. When inhaled, the oil eliminates the feeling of hunger pangs hence proper adherence to the set feeding schedule.

It is important to note that before using the essential oils for weight loss, it is advisable to consult your nutritionist, gym instructor or a physician if on other medication especially for long term illnesses.

Conclusion

Weight loss is a topic that hits an individual at a point in their lives. It is difficult to lose weight and many have resulted to harmful chemicals that lead to weight loss but leaving the body with a host of side effects to deal with. The essential oils boost the weight loss being achieved through use of healthy diet and exercise without causing side effects to the body. This makes them the best natural solution for weight loss.

Essential Oils for Common Ailments

Essential oils are among the most effective alternative medicine for common ailments. These medicinal oils are facilitates for natural body healing process. This is because they do not contain any chemical components that bring about manipulation of the immune system of the body while posing serious undesirable effects to the individual. In this case, one does not have to make use of prescribed medications as the oils works marvelously even for the diagnosed diseases. These oils do not only bring about healing as many other processed medicines do but they are the best in boosting the immunity in the body to resist most of the common ailments that attack the body. In this way, they keep the body healthy. Here are the most amazing essential oils effective for treatment of some common ailments.

Irritating cough

Essential oils provide good results in the treatment of an irritating cough. Everyone has had an experience of a cough that is persistent and knows how irritating this can be. The cough attacks children as well as adults sometimes making it impossible to sleep at night or to complete important tasks. Some of the essential oils are natural cough suppressants that act through inhalation, when applied topically or swallowed into the body, getting rid of the cough completely within a short period of use. They include;

- *Eucalyptus Radiata Oil*

  This is an essential oil that eliminates a cough when applied topically or as an inhalant. The natural oil preparation cause a soothing effect while clearing the respiratory tract hence making breathing easy. This essential oil derived from eucalyptus plants treats coughs, unblocks the respiratory system and relieves an irritated throat bringing back wellness and comfort to the individual.

- *On Guard Protective Blend oil*

  This essential oil is prepared to diffuse in the air as well as act in the body's internal organs. The preparation is safe on the people who are not having any symptoms when inhaled. On guard protective blend is diffused into the air within the room where it clears all the disease causing agents such as virus, fungi and bacteria. When taken into the body, this essential oil boosts the immune system hence fighting the current infection that is bringing about the cough while protecting the body from farther attacks. It is important to note that a cough is highly contagious meaning that it can be spread fast from one person to the next. On guard protective blend should be dissolved into the air to stop the spread of colds and influenza that results in persistent irritating coughs.

- *Breathe Respiratory Blend oil*

    Among the top cough suppressants essential oils is the breath respiratory blend oil. It acts topically and when diffused into the air it soothes the neck and chest hence clearing the respiratory tract, especially the sinuses and lungs as well. It also helps in ensuring a sound sleep when having the flu accompanied by a cough.

Skin rashes

Skin rashes can occur in any part of the body as a result of direct contact with harmful chemicals, common allergens such as some leaves or plant sap, insect stings or bites and infections. This leads to redness of the area, patches and sometimes it is accompanied by itching and irritation. The essential oils provide the best remedies for skin rashes and irritation leading to a smooth healthy skin quickly. Some of the best essential oil formulas for skin conditions are;

- *Lavender Essential oil*

    This essential oil preparation is applied topically to facilitate local healing on the skin. This oil is ideal for treatment of superficial burns, bruises and blisters on the skin. When applied soon after an insect bite or sting, it brings about the desired soothing effect that prevents skin irritation. It is safe to use on irritated lips.

- *Roman Chamomile oil*

    This amazing essential oil is derived from the chamomile plant. It is highly effective for treatment of varying skin conditions caused by allergy or infection such as boils, itchy rashes, skin inflammation, acne and eczema. When applied topically, the preparation causes a soothing effect on the skin to eliminate irritation giving way to development of new skin.

- *Melaleuca or Tea Tree oil*

    Melaleuca is a topical preparation form of essential oil which is effective for treatment of rashes on the skin and effects of athlete's foot condition. It also helps the skin to regenerate, becoming healthy and smooth.

Severe back pain

Severe back pain can be caused by strain after carrying heavy luggage or excessive exercises. In addition, back pains can be as a result of underlying gynecological or spine issues. Spine related conditions can lead to excruciating pain in the back. Here are essential oils that offer relief from such pain.

- *Cypress oil*

    Cypress is an essential oil that is prepared specifically for topical application. The mode of action of this oil is to relax tightened and tense muscles in the body. When applied on the back region this essential oil leads to increased blood flow around the region hence relaxation of the muscles. This helps in eliminating the spasms and cramps experienced in the muscles.

- *Deep Blue Soothing Blend oil*

Deep blue soothing blend is an essential oil derived from a combination of natural substances. This essential oil is made effective due to the presence of peppermint, osmanthus and camphor. The oil also contains chamomile from Germany, Helichrysum, blue tansy and wintergreen. When applied to the muscles on the back they soothe the pain and eliminate tiredness and muscle tension after exercise. The oil preparation provides deep tissue massage which is therapeutic for different back conditions.

Stomach issues

It is not healthy to rush for over counter medication every time there is stomach related issues. The following essential oils are effective in getting rid of stomach and digestive related issues.

- *Digestzen Digestive Blend Oil*

This essential oil acts both locally and internally. In case of abdominal discomfort as a result of digestive related issues, nausea and motion sickness the preparation should be rubbed on the tummy leading to relief. It can also be taken with main meals to aid in digestion hence preventing stomach issues. In order to make digestion effective in children, the digestzen essential oil should be rubbed on the sole of the feet.

- *Peppermint Oil*

This essential oil is effective in the treatment of nausea and other related digestive issues. In the case of irritable bowel syndrome, colic and excessive gas in the stomach the peppermint oil should be taken orally or applied on the tummy.

- *Ginger Essential Oil*

Ginger is among the essential oils that are effective for treatment of abdominal cramps, diarrhea, vomiting and excessive gas in the stomach. It can be taken orally or applied on the tummy region to relieve discomfort.

Conclusion

Essential oils have a long history in treatment of different ailments in the human body. They can be taken orally, applied topically or used as aerosols to bring about the desired effects. They are natural preparations that are derived from plants that grow naturally in the forests and gardens. However, accurate diagnosis of the ailment is essential for successful treatment with essential oils.

TOP WAYS TO USE ESSENTIAL OILS AROUND THE HOME

Essential oils provide the best natural treatment for varying ailments as they are derived from plants. These plant extracts are pure and highly concentrated to give the desired results for specific ailments. These oils are extracted from the particular plants through steam distillation and pressure process. Once the essential oils are fully processed, they are comfortable to use as they do not lead to any adverse reactions or any other undesirable effects to the body. In addition, the oils have a good scent hence ideal to use on the skin. Their healing potential makes them essential for use by all and around the home for different purposes.

In order to maintain their potency it is important to understand that they require good storage as their shelf life is quite short. When using them around the home, they should be stored in cool dry places and away from sunlight. If stored under those conditions, the oils can stay fresh with their full therapeutic potential for some years. However, the essential oils derived from the citrus plant should not be preserved for more than one year. This is because the oils do not contain any preservatives as other medications do.

What are uses of the essential oils at home?

Room disinfectants

The essential oils are ideal for use as room disinfectants at home. They can be used to disinfect the room in which a sick person with a contagious infection such as the flu is living. Some of the oils, such as the on guard protective blend and lemon essential oils are dissolved into the air killing the disease causing organisms within the room. This helps in preventing transmission of the air borne infection from the infected person to others who frequent the room.

Home air freshener

There are numerous air fresheners in the market today but unfortunately many are prepared with chemicals that add toxins into the body when inhaled. The best option is to have the essential oils and spraying little sparks into the stuffy rooms for freshness. The essential oil air freshener sprays are natural with a nice scent that makes the room fresh all day long.

Daily baths

The essential oils offer the best aromatherapy to the body. This leads to relaxation of the muscles while getting rid of the stress in the entire body. The oils give one an opportunity to enjoy time in the bathtub each day. The best essential oils for taking a bath are the ones with chamomile and lavender, especially after a tiring and long day. In addition, the pine oils as well as the rosemary essential oils are ideal for those engaged in regular workout as they help in toning of the muscles when used for a whole body soak after extensive exercise.

Spray to keep rodents off

Essential oils sprays are the best solution for farm home owners in handling rodent problems. Mice being the most common type of rodents that invade the private space in the house, the Peppermint oils direct them out of the house within no time. This spray is user friendly while hard on the mice making it safe to use in the house. It is easy to prepare the spray by adding about two teaspoons of the peppermint oil into a cup of water and sprinkling or spraying with a hand sprayer in the areas that are likely to be inhabited by the mouse. This can also be sprayed in the food stores as the oil does not contaminate the food substances since it does not contain any chemicals.

Beauty body scrub

Rough skin makes one uncomfortable as it changes the appearance of an individual. This is common with people living in areas that experience harsh winter weather. Instead of getting body scrubs derived from chemicals that can react with the skin, it advisable to have a natural body scrub made of essential oils extracted from the plants. These oil body scrubs exfoliate the dry and rough skin making it soft, smooth and bright. They also provide the required scent to keep the body fresh and rejuvenated hence looking young.

Body deodorants

The essential oils products have a fragrance that is fresh and nice. This makes the ideal deodorants for the daily use. This keeps one fresh and without any traces of the body odor while getting rid of the worry about skin irritation or respiratory system allergies.

Kitchen wash detergents

The essential oils acts as the best detergents to be used in the kitchen. The kitchen is the most sensitive area in the house as food substances are prepared in there with high likelihood of contamination that can result in serious stomach issues. This can be avoided by making use of the essential oils that not only clean the target areas such as the kitchen benches and utensils but also disinfects the entire kitchen. This ensures the health of the entire family. In case of disinfecting the utensils, the lemon essential oils can be used whereby the oily and dirty utensils are soaked in hot water with the right concentration of the oil for some minutes then cleaning is done.

Feet soak

The soles of the feet are prone to build up of dead skin hence becoming rough. The essential oils are ideal for a foot soak, that leads to softening of the dead rough skin on the sole of the feet. Later, the same oils can be used to scrub off the skin leaving the feet clean, soft and smooth naturally.

Cleaning the toys

Babies are sensitive to dirt as their immune system is not fully developed. When kids are playing with toys, they place them on the surfaces and on the floor where they collect dirt. The same toys are put in the mouth while playing hence a good source of disease causing organisms. Therefore, the toys need to be cleaned every day with the disinfectant essential oils in order to eliminate the pathogens present. Soaking the toys in hot water with the essential oils helps in effectively making them clean and germ free.

Conclusion

Essential oils provide all round health and wellness in a household. This is because with, at least, a set of five oils in the house, the chances for infection are minimized as the oils acts as disinfectants in the house when they are used as air fresheners and cleaning agents. The oils protect the skin from infections while softening it and keeping it smooth when used as beauty products and when added into the bathing shampoo. The essential oils are also taken orally with water and fluids, inhaled or rubbed on the skin to bring about natural healing.

ESSENTIAL OILS FOR BABIES AND CHILDREN

Aromatherapy by use of essential oils is good for the whole family including babies. There are many ailments that affect the babies and small children that can be healed or prevented by use of the natural oils. However, it should be remembered that though the essential oils are natural and pure, they are also highly concentrated. This can be strong for newborn babies and children as well. This is because the systems in the body of babies and children are not adequately developed, thus they might not process the oils, especially those that are taken orally or inhaled. In addition, it is important to consult a pediatrician for accurate diagnosis as babies and some small children cannot express exactly where the pain or discomfort is in their body.

Precaution when using the essential oils on babies and children

Taking caution should not discourage you from using the essential oils on young children and babies. These are measures that should be taken when administering the oils to the young one to keep them safe.

Dilute the essential oil

When using the essential oils for babies and children, it is advisable to dilute them with vegetable oil. In this case, 1 to 3 drops should be dissolved in about ½ or one teaspoon of oil for the oils that are to be taken orally. When using the oil to bath, the oil should be mixed with the baby's bath gel but in a small quantity. This makes the oils dilute enough for the baby to digest and for it to be gentle on the fragile skin.

Identify the safe essential oils for babies

It is important to identify the safe essential oils to be used by babies and small children. This is because some of the oils might have a flavor or scent that is too strong for the baby to bear. For example the peppermint essential oils might not be ideal for babies as they can cause a burning sensation when ingested, rubbed on the body skin or inhaled. Therefore, it is advisable to research or enquire from an expert the oils that are safe for the babies and young children.

Keep essential oils out of children's reach

Just like any other substances, the essential oils should be kept away from babies and children's reach. It should be remembered that though the oils are natural and pure, excess of everything is poisonous. Therefore, the oils should be locked in the cabinet in which the medications for the family are kept. In case the baby or child ingests any of the essential oil by mistake, urgent action should be taken as it is difficult to know the amount of the oil swallowed. In this case, the child should be given liquids that are oil soluble, that includes milk or cream. One can give any of the two or mix the cream and milk and give to the child to drink.

Avoid mixing essential oils

When using essential oils for children and babies, one type of oil should be used at a time. Mixing of different types of the oils to be given at once is discouraged as the mixture might be very strong for the babies. The ideal way is to make use of a single oil for a period of time especially for bathing the baby. However, the oils to be inhaled or taken orally should be given when need arises or occasionally for boosting immunity of the babies.

Consult pediatrician

A pediatrician should be consulted before using the essential oils on newborn babies and children below the age of two. This is aimed at determining the amount of the oil to be given to the baby according to the specific age and for the right diagnosis in case of an ailment. This helps in keeping the babies and children safe while ensuring good health.

Different conditions and essential oils for babies and children

Different conditions and ailments in babies and children can be prevented and healed by use of essential oils. This eliminates chances of exposing the babies and young children to over the counter medications for every light ailment as this can lead to resistance, especially in antibiotics. Here are different conditions or ailments in babies and children that requires the use of essential oils.

Constipation

Constipation is common in newborn babies and children when whining is being done. This is because their digestive system at this stage is not used to digesting the breast milk and ingested food substances respectively. This can also result when children are introduced to semi-solid food substances without providing adequate fluids for the child to drink. In order to prevent or eliminate constipation, orange, mandarin, rosemary and ginger based essential oils should be used as they are effective and safe on babies and children.

Diaper rash and dry skin

Babies and children are prone to diaper rash and dry skin. This makes the babies irritable and uncomfortable. In this case, roman chamomile or lavender oil should be mixed with any of the vegetable oil and applied on the areas affected by the rash. Sandal and rosewood oils are ideal for a dry skin as they moisturize it keeping it soft and smooth.

Fever and flu

Fever is the first manifestation of ailment in babies and children. Thus, before rushing the baby to the hospital for treatment it is important to handle the fever first by diluting lavender essential oil in vegetable oil and applying it behind the ears, under the feet and the back of the neck of the baby. If the baby or the child is suffering from a cold, it is advisable to use diluted lemon or cypress oils to bathe the baby.

Colic in babies

Colic is very common in newborn babies and children as they get adapted to the new diet. The Ylang

Ylang, mandarin, Bergamot, Roman Chamomile, ginger and Marjoram can be used. Any of the selected essential oils should be dissolved in almond oil and then applied on the baby's stomach.

Conclusion

Essential oils are effective and safe on babies and children. Caution should be taken in order to ensure the safety of the babies and small children whose baby organs are not yet fully developed to function adequately. However, if the baby has been born premature but discharged from hospital, the essential oils should only be used at the age of two years and above.

ESSENTIAL OILS IN REDUCING ANXIETY, STRESS AND DEPRESSION

Essential oils are effective in handling issues related to anxiety, stress and depression. Anxiety, stress and depression are grouped among the most disturbing and debilitating emotional and physiological responses to the stimuli within the surrounding environment. When these conditions are constant in a person's life, they result to other serious complications that include heart disease, diabetes, asthma, gastrointestinal issues and obesity. One can put in measures to stay away from stressful situations that bring about anxiety and depression. However, this has resulted in more tension in most of the cases due to the presence of stressors or some inherited traits that makes one prone to stress.

Essential oils play an important role in eliminating the above conditions by bringing about calmness and emotional balance in an individual. The effects of the oils are sustained when used on daily basis by the individual and around the house bringing about emotional wellness. They can be applied topically on the skin, inhaled, taken with food and drinks or used in different ways within the house.

Effective essential oils for treatment of anxiety, stress and depression

Citrus Sinensis or Orange Essential Oil

This is among the essential oils whose fragrances help in handling anxiety and stress effectively. When the fragrance of the orange oil gets into the body system it brings a sense of calmness and deep peace that empowers one's mind to be more positive. This essential oil is also known for its role in boosting the immunity system in the person's body. This leads to health and wellness for the previously suffering person.

Blue Tansy oil

The blue tansy essential oil is known for its ability to calm the nerves hence neutralizing the feelings of anger and other negative emotions that leads to deep anxiety, stress and depression. The oil is best used when dissolved in a liquid such as water or tea.

Ylang Ylang oil

Ylang Ylang is one of the potent essential oils that enhance relaxation of mind, body and soul of an individual. This natural oil acts on the body cells in order to bring about emotional equilibrium hence building confidence, deep peace and a sense of wellness. This eliminates anxiety, stress and depression.

Tangerine natural oil

The tangerine essential oil acts on the nerves and brain thus making the person calm with reduced anxiety and stress. Its action is facilitated by the presence of aldehydes and ester in it, that also causes some sedation effects in a person hence ensuring a deep calm sleep. When one has had a restful night sleep, the triggers of stress, anxiety and depression are stopped thus preventing the negative emotional conditions.

Patchouli oil

This essential oil leads to relaxation by causing sedative effects in an individual. This helps the person to calm down while eliminating insomnia. A good sleep helps an individual to recover from stress, anxiety and depression and gets them waking up with renewed energy.

How to make best use of the above essential oils

The essential oils for treatment of anxiety, stress and depression related ailments can be used in different ways. This entails the route of administration for them to provide the desired results in the body of an individual bringing about calmness, relaxation, peace of mind and positive emotions. Here are different ways of using the natural oils;

Application topically

This refers to making use of the essential oils by applying them on different parts of the skin. In order to treat or prevent anxiety, stress and depression it is advisable to apply the selected oil on the soles of the feet, around the wrist and at the back of the neck. This should be done after a warm bath every morning to bring about calmness and positive emotions as well as in the evening for a relaxed and sound night's sleep.

Internal administration

The essential oils can be administered internally in order to act on the internal body systems. In this case, the individual who is prone to anxiety, stress and depression should inhale any of the oils regularly during the day and before going to bed. Also, the selected oils can be taken together with the meals while dissolved in water or tea. This helps in stimulating the internal organs to function adequately while acting on the brain and nerve cells that help in calming the individual down. This eliminates the tension and negative emotions that lead to emotional imbalance.

As an air freshener

Once an individual is diagnosed with emotional or psychological challenges, it is advisable to make use of the essential oils as air freshener. Here, the oils can be sprayed in the house, car and the office to provide a cool aroma in the entire environment. This helps the individual to stay calm with positive emotions throughout the day and night. For best results, one can choose to spray different essential oils interchangeably after every three to four hours. This brings about change, not getting used to only one fragrance as there is high possibility of the body becoming insensitive to that particular type of essential oil.

Dissolved in bathtub

Dissolving the essential oils in the bathtub provides amazing results in the treatment and prevention of anxiety, stress and depression related conditions. Whether prone to emotional imbalances or not, one would agree that after a long stressful day what is needed is a warm long soak in the bathtub. Well, this experience is fortified by dissolving the essential oils into the warm water and soaking in it for as long as one needs to. This method can be combined with other modes of using the essential oils for desired results.

Conclusion

Essential oils have proven to be highly effective in treatment and prevention of anxiety, stress and depression in both human beings and pets. One can make use of different types of oils at different times of the day in order to achieve that positive energy and emotions all the time. Essential oils have a long history of bringing about a feeling of calmness, deep peace, sound sleep and relaxation; eliminating emotional imbalances that results in stress, anxiety and depression.

HOW TO GET BEST ESSENTIAL OILS AND USE

Essential oils are available in the market sold in different brands. They are effective for prevention and healing of varying ailments in both human persons and pets. In addition, the oils enhance beauty while slowing the aging process by acting on the skin of an individual. Essential oils are extracted from specific plants through distillation process. The extracts are processed without mixing with other chemicals that might be harmful to human body. Thus, the oils are packed while pure and highly concentrated ready for use as a preventive or healing agent in a person's body. These oils are also used at home for various purposes such as disinfectants, insect repellants, air fresheners, for pets and bath.

Due to the availability of different brands in the market being traded by varying providers it is important to compare the brands of essential oils. In this case, it is advisable to base the comparison on the need at hand, quality and the cost of the oil. This helps in identifying the best brand that is effective for the ailment or for other purposes. In order to get the oils with therapeutic properties, it is important to distinguish between the fragrance oils and essential oils. When the right oil has been identified, the mixing should be done well for best results.

The process of comparing essential oils

Identify the need at hand

In order to choose the right essential oils, it is important to identify the need at hand. This refers to the purpose the oils are required for. This helps in coming up with a list of the oils that are likely to serve the purpose.

Check on the properties of each brand

When comparing the essential oils for the specific purpose, it is advisable to check on the properties of each brand. This entails getting the information on what the oil can do in the body, establishing if it is highly effective for the intended purpose. This aids in identifying the oil that works best in achieving the desired results.

Compare the quality and cost

There are different essential oil providers in the online market trading in the same products. However, they differ significantly in terms of quality and cost. Thus, browse through the websites of the essential oils providers and have access to the customer's reviews. This helps in getting to know their history in providing high quality oils. After the right oil brands and best providers are identified, one should request for a quote from at least three to four providers for the oils to be purchased. The quotes help in comparing the prices from different providers.

The difference between the fragrance oils and essential oils

When searching for the best essential oils it is important to differentiate between the fragrance and essential oils. This is because it is easy to confuse the two but their effects on the body are different. Here are the differences between the two;

Therapeutic properties

The essential oils have therapeutic properties while the fragrance oils do not have. This means that the essential oils protect and heal the body from varying ailments while the fragrance oils have no healing effects in both human beings and pets.

The source

The source for the two types of oils differs significantly. The essential oils are derived from plants hence the source of their therapeutic properties and scent. On the other hand, the fragrance oils are artificially made and scented. The source of the essential oils makes them natural and pure compared to the fragrance oils that are artificial.

Purpose

The purpose for the essential oils differs from that of the fragrance oils. This is because the essential oils are used as disinfectants, insect repellants, and treatment for various ailments as well as anti-aging and beauty products. On the other side, the fragrance oils are used as air fresheners and insect repellants.

Mode of preparation

The essential oils are extracted from the plants and then packaged as pure natural oils. In this case, the provider is required to indicate the list of ingredients present in the oil. This helps the consumers know the effects of the oils purchased. Fragrance oils on their part are artificially prepared in the laboratory. Though they contain an essential oil in low quantities, other artificial ingredients are added. In addition, the provider is not required to provide the list of the ingredients hence caution should be taken as they may contain ingredients that reacts with an individual.

How to mix essential oils for use

There are some specific conditions that require specific mixture of essential oils for desired results. Here are mixture samples of essential oils for various needs.

Essential oils for headaches

When preparing essential oils for healing headaches, it is advisable to establish the cause of the headache. This can be due to stress related conditions, infections or trauma. In any case, the oil blend derived from calendula flowers and olive oil should be mixed. Here, one teaspoon of the calendula flower should be added into the olive oil. Also, 1 drop of the peppermint essential oil can be added to boost the effect. Once the mixture is ready, it should be rubbed at the back of the neck thus relieving the headache.

Essential oils for menstrual cramps

Menstrual cramps are common in women within the child bearing age bracket. The cramps are characterized by pain in the lower abdominal region, numbness of the thighs, nausea and sometimes vomiting. In order to relieve this pain, 5 drops of lavender oil, 15 drops of peppermint oil and cypress oil about 10 drops should be added in the almond or any other carrier oil. They should be stirred till adequately mixed. Then, the even mixture should be rubbed or used to massage the lower abdominal region. This can be repeated three times in a day for the best results.

Essential oils for stress and depression

Stress and depression affects the emotional faculty of an individual. These are conditions that are related and they make one unable to cope with daily challenges. They also lead to a lack of energy to carryout daily tasks due to lack of positive thinking and energy. In order to relieve the negative emotions and make the body relax, the grapefruit, Ylang Ylang and Jasmine essential oils should be used along with Epsom salt. Here, about 15 drops of Ylang Ylang and those of Jasmine should be added into 45 drops of grapefruit of oil and then mixed with around 2-3 cups of Epsom salt. Once the mixture is ready, one should use it for bathing at least twice in a day.

Conclusion

Essential oils should be selected and mixed carefully in order to provide the desired results. If one is to mix different types, the oils to be used together should have the properties that cause the required effects in order to heal the existing ailment. Enough information should be gathered from the websites of essential oils experts available online.

TIPS ON MAKING ESSENTIAL OILS AND FACTS ON AROMATHERAPY

It is important to understand some facts about aromatherapy in order make the essential oils. There is no difference between aromatherapy and essential oils. The fact is that the aromatherapy entails making use of essential oils which are extracted from plants. Through the process of aromatherapy, the essential oils brings about healing while preventing infections by killing the germs. The essential oils are also effective as cleaning agents, for use on pets and as deodorants.

How essential oils work in aromatherapy

- During an aromatherapy session, the particular essential oils are inhaled directly or sprayed, massaged on the body muscles and ingested when dissolved in water or tea. The essential oils are easily absorbed into the skin and lungs due to their tiny aromatic molecules hence providing the desired results. When inhaled, the essential oils bring about healing from the common cold and flu that is leading to congestion in the chest and nasal region while inducing an irritating cough. The essential oils clear the chest and sinuses while soothing the cough and suppressing it.

- In addition, the small molecules of the essential oils used gets into the bloodstream and are circulated in different organs where they boost the body's natural immunity and heal the existing diseases. When applied on the skin, the essential oils penetrate the different layers of the skin moisturizing, smoothening and softening it. Also, the oils acts on the skin straightening the wrinkles and fine lines present while gradually slowing down the aging process. In this way, they become effective recipes for aromatherapy for beauty purposes and as anti-aging agents, as they keep the skin naturally beautiful and young.

- Essential oils are also effective for treatment of pet related ailments. They are safe for use on pets through inhalation and ingesting when mixed with water. The oils maintain health in pets when they are mixed with the shampoo for bathing the pets. In this case, the oils act as disinfectants and health enhancing agents.

How to save on essential oils cost

The cost of essential oils is not only evaluated using the cumulative price but checking on their quality and potency. This is because the essential oils are natural and pure and give the desired results without causing adverse reactions on the body systems. In addition, the oils last for long time, as just few drops are required in each single use regardless of the mode of administration as they are highly concentrated.

Therefore, when buying the essential oils, it is important to consider the following;

- Identify a reliable provider in order to get the original essential oils.

- Compare different providers and evaluate the type of essential oils they have to offer.

- Request a quote from several best providers in order to compare costs and settle for the one with the highest quality oils at the best rates in the market.

Tips on making essential oils

The source of essential oils is basically herbs and plants growing naturally in farms and forests. The oils are derived from specific plants or herbs through the process of distillation. This makes the oils ready for use on human beings, pets and for cleaning purposes. One can use the essential oils for the majority of household tasks as cleaning agents, air fresheners and disinfectants. If you have access to particular herbs and plants that are sources of essential oils, you can make the oils at home. Here are some tips that you can follow for a successful process;

- *Identify the right source*

   The first step in the making of the essential oils at home is the identification of the right source of the desired oil. This entails locating the plant or herb that you will use to extract the oil. This can be from a forest or a farm. In case you are planning to make different types of the oils, then the various types of plants and herbs should be identified.

- *Collect the right part*

   In order to make the essential oils successfully, it is important to know the part of the plant to be used. Here, you need to have the right information about the part of the herb or plant that is a good source of the oil. This can be the stem, leaves or roots of the plant. Thus, collect the parts in adequate quantities to make the required amount of oils.

- *Mix the herbs or plant with carrier oil*

The mixing of herbs or plants with the selected carrier oils is the beginning of the process of making the essential oils. At this stage, the carrier oil such as the olive oil should be mixed with the required amount of the herb or plant from which to extract the oil from. The recommended amount of the herb or plant to be used should be ¼ cup. The olive and herbs or plants should be mixed evenly in a medium pot.

- *Heat the mixture*

Once the olive oil and the ¼ cup of plants or herbs are well mixed, it is the time to heat them. There are two ways of heating the mixture. You can heat the mixture of the herbs and oil in an oven set at low heat. However, you need to check the amount of heat as it should be maintained as low as possible. Alternatively, you can place the mixture in a glass jar and let it to heat under the sun. You should leave the mixture to simmer for about five and six hours.

- *Strain and package the essential oil*

This is the last stage in making the essential oils. Here, you need to get an unbleached cheese cloth in order to get oils that are pure. Then, sieve out the herbs or plant contents from the olive oil while pouring the contents in a glass jar. Remember that the essential oils are sensitive to light and warm temperatures. Thus, pack the produced essential oils into a dark amber jar and close it tightly. Then store the essential oils in a cool, dry and dark place.

Conclusion

In order to have successful aromatherapy that brings about healing, health and beauty by use of essential oils, it is important to observe the proper making process as well as the right way of buying the oil. This helps in getting high quality, pure and highly concentrated oils that provide the desired results in aromatherapy. It is advisable to consult an essential oils expert for adequate information if need be.

FREQUENTLY ASKED QUESTIONS ON ESSENTIAL OILS

The essential oils have become popular in the recent past for use in human beings, pets and household tasks due to their amazing results in healing, protecting the body from infections and beauty effects while slowing down the aging process in a person. However, several questions ring in many people's mind especially in the process of making decisions on whether to make use of the oils or not. Here are the frequently asked questions and possible answers that can help in making an informed decision on the use of essential oils.

Are the essential oils safe for use on babies and children?

The essential oils are safe for use on children beyond two years. However, they can be used on babies but caution should be taken by diluting few drops of the oils in the ideal carrier oils such as the almond or olive oil. A pediatrician should be consulted before using the oils on babies especially the newborn babies for guidance.

Can I use essential oils for my pet care?

Absolutely yes! Essential oils are effective on different pets. They can be used in disinfecting the pet house, utensils and beddings. In addition, you can mix few drops of oils with water or other fluids intended to be given to the pets to enhance natural healing process. When bathing the pet, the oils can be added into the pets' shampoo for a healthy and parasite free fur and skin.

Is it possible to make essential oils at home?

Essential oils can be made at home through the distillation method. This is a simple process if the herbs and plants required for different types of oils are readily available. Adequate information on the process can be access online.

Do essential oils expire or can they be used until a bottle is empty?

Essential oils do expire after a period of time, that varies from one type of oil to another. It is important to note that these oils are sensitive as they do not contain any preservatives. Most of the oils last between 6-12 months with others having a shelf life of beyond one year. One needs to check the expiry date indicated on the bottle by the manufacturer.

Are the essential oils safe for use in pregnancy?

Well, essential oils are generally safe especially when used under the cover of carrier oils. However, it is advisable to consult the gynecologist or a physician before using the essential oils especially in the first trimester of pregnancy.

Since essential oils are highly concentrated, should I dilute them using water?

It is true that the essential oils are highly concentrated. They are only diluted when being used on children and young pets as their body systems are not well developed to process high concentrated oils. In this case, the oils should be diluted using the carrier oils such as almond oils. When using the oils orally, a few drops can be added into the tea or water but in the right proportions.

Is there a relationship between the essential oils and fragrance oils?

A relationship exists between the essential oils and fragrance oils. This is because the fragrance oils contain an essential oil but in very low levels. However, they both differ significantly as fragrance oils are artificially processed in the laboratories hence not natural and they do not contain any healing or antimicrobial properties. The essential oils on the other hand are derived from plants so they are natural and pure. They also contain antibiotic, antimicrobial, healing and analgesic properties.

My skin is getting wrinkled at a high rate, should I have any hope in essential oils?

Wrinkles and fine lines appear on the skin due to escalating aging process in an individual. You can slow down the aging process by making use of essential oils regularly. You can consider adding few drops of essential oils in the bathing shampoo, taking them with water or tea and applying them on the skin as beauty products. The essential oils straighten the wrinkled skin and moisturize it hence appearing young and attractive.

Do I need to buy essential oils in large quantities?

Well, the quantity of the essential oils to be bought depends on the need. However, the oils are usually concentrated so only a little measure is required each time.

Are the essential oils natural?

The natural oils are 100% natural without any traces of chemicals in them. They are derived from naturally growing herbs and plants. The oils are extracted through a natural process known as distillation.

If I use the essential oils as part of my beauty products, will they bleach my skin?

The fact that the essential oils are pure and natural mean they do not have any bleaching effects on the skin. When used on the skin for a period of time, it makes the skin smooth, soft and well toned hence enhancing natural beauty and making the skin to glow.

Can the essential oils be used for menstrual cramps?

Yes, the essential oils are very effective on menstrual cramps. They should be rubbed on the lower abdominal region at least thrice in a day to provide prolonged relief from the cramps.

I am looking for a chemical free air freshener for my house, can I use essential oils?

It is advisable to make use of essential oils based air fresheners as they do not contain any chemicals that can contaminate the air leading to allergies and other complications. The essential oil air fresheners also offers protection from airborne infections as they have antimicrobial properties.

Is depression controlled by use of essential oils?

The essential oils acts on the brain and nerve cells leading to relaxation. In addition, the oils stimulate the brain resulting to a sense of calmness in an individual while inducing sleep. This helps in eliminating anxiety, stress and depressive moods.

Conclusion

The essential oils have aroma molecules that release the desired scent. They also contain antimicrobial, antibacterial and vitamins that are vital in boosting the natural immunity in the body, killing germs and bringing about healing for various ailments.

So that's it! Thank you for taking the time to read my book. I hope you enjoyed this short read and find it very informative. Essential oils are prepared to ensure all round health and wellbeing in the entire family. They are available in the beauty and natural alternative treatment stores both offline in the USA and online worldwide. They are safe to use without any adverse reactions that can result in serious health complications or body harm. In addition, in the wake of rising resistance to the over the counter drugs due to self medication and abuse, the essential oils are the way to go for a natural safe process. Again, thank you for taking the time to inform yourself about essential oils. Please don't forget to leave me a review!

CONTENTS